Walking

for Weight Loss

Get Fit, Feel Great, and Look Amazing

Sam Hignett

Table of Contents

Introduction

Walking is a great way to start your exercise regime for anyone looking to improve their health and fitness. What can be easier than stepping out of your front door and walking your way to a better, healthier, and a happier you.

Walking is something we all do every day even if it's just walking to the end of the road for some groceries, so turning our daily walking routines into workouts takes very little effort but produces fantastic results for our overall health. Just a few more steps and you will have benefits that will last you a lifetime!

This book contains proven steps and strategies on how to start a walking exercise program that can help you in many ways, including helping to increase your fitness, help you to lose weight, or by helping you to use walking as a way to relax and unwind. Walking just has so many benefits!

This book also looks at numerous aspects that you can use to help improve your walking experience including equipment guidelines, warm up routines, a 10 000 step walking programme and the importance of the correct cool down procedures.

If you have never been an avid walker, this book will tell you everything you need to know to prepare you for the joy of walking.

Go on, walk yourself to a healthier, fitter, sleeker you!

Thanks again for buying this book, I hope you enjoy it!

Chapter 1 – The Health Benefits

of Walking

As we all know, exercise is good for us and walking is perhaps the easiest form of exercise we can undertake. It does not need any fancy equipment, bar a pair of good shoes and can be undertaken at any time. Walking also has numerous benefits for us.

Recent studies in the UK, conducted by the Ramblers and Macmillan cancer support group, have shown that walking can help save many lives each year, in fact, the figures suggest around 37 000. Exercise is also extremely necessary in the fight against obesity and type 2 diabetes.

Of course, walking has many other health benefits. Let's take a look at a few of them in closer detail.

Walking helps to reduce body fat

A good walk is a great way to reduce body fat. This is especially useful to people who are obese and often cannot do another form of exercise. Although walking can be difficult in the beginning, slowly building both the distance and speed at which you walk will help to reduce body fat over time and will lead to weight loss.

How exactly does it do this? Well, although walking is a fairly low impact workout, it still helps to increase both heart rate and breathing rates, which will slowly build cardiovascular fitness. This will also increase your overall endurance and boost energy levels.

Walking is an extremely effective exercise for people who carry too much belly fat. This form of fat is particularly dangerous and can lead to heart disease and type 2 diabetes. These fat stores are the first to be used as a form of energy by your body whenever a decent session of cardiovascular exercise takes place.

Of course, your should walk as briskly as your body allows. This ensures that you gain the full benefit and fat loss potential from a good workout. Walking can burn between 300 to 400 calories per hour, depending on your fitness level and current weight.

Walking helps to control blood glucose levels

Exercise is a great way to help your body control the way it processes and uses glucose. Even a moderate walk can help your muscles use glucose more effectively, often by up to 20 times when compared to a resting state. This is extremely important in obese people who might be on the verge of type 2 diabetes.

Walking helps to reduce the risk of heart disease

As we get older, we are at risk of heart disease. This is true of people who are obese, especially around the belly region. Walking can help to protect against many heart problems. One of the main ways it does this is by lowering Low-density lipoprotein cholesterol levels which we will explore a little later in this chapter.

As an aerobic exercise, walking helps to raise your heart rate, improves blood circulation, helps to lower blood pressure, reduces the probability of blood clots and ultimately helps to make your heart a stronger organ.

Walking helps to fight against Alzheimer's disease

By walking each day, the brain releases a number of chemicals that aid with memory and learning. These chemicals also help to fight brain degeneration that begins to occur naturally in the middle 40's. Although walking or exercise cannot prevent Alzheimer's, they are important factors in fighting its degenerative effects on the brain.

Walking helps in the fight against certain cancers

A study by the American Cancer Association has shown that walking for an hour a day lowers the risk of breast cancer in woman by 14%. Studies have also shown that exercise helps our bodies process food quicker, meaning that it travels faster through our colon, reducing the risk of any toxins being absorbed into our bodies.

Walking helps to raise metabolism levels

Exercise is the best way to raise your body's metabolic rate, helping to ensure that it continues to burn calories long after the exertion has ended. A good walk can raise your metabolism for a full two hours after completion.

Of course, as you get fitter, your metabolism increases and burns excess fats stores more easily. Walking also can help to control hormone levels in your body.

Walking helps to control cholesterol levels

Low-density lipoprotein or bad cholesterol often can build up due to lack of exercise and weight gain. This form of cholesterol is often associated with a large increase in the risk of heart disease.

By walking and exercising, your body moves this cholesterol to the liver, where it is processed into bile and either excreted or used in the digestive process.

Walking leads to stronger bones

Walking, along with the correct intake of calcium, helps to increase the strength of your skeleton. This is a particular benefit to females who may suffer from osteoporosis in later life.

Walking is good for mental health

Exercise is a brilliant way to help improve mental health and to lift our spirits. It can also benefit us in numerous other ways including:

- Reducing stress: Walking can help to raise the levels of nonrepinephrine in your brain. This chemical controls how your brain reacts to stressful situations. With a raised concentration of nonrepinephrine, stress is not only reduced, but your body's ability to deal with it is enhanced as well.

- Improved mood: Walking is a perfect way to feel happier! As we exercise, various endorphins are released into our system. These help to improve our mood. Exercise is also an excellent way to fight both anxiety and depression.

- Increase brainpower and improve memory: Walking, as well as other exercise, promotes the creation of new brain cells which helps to improve our overall mental performance including memory and learning.

Walking is good for relaxation

Nothing beats the feeling of coming home after a long, strenuous walk. Not only does it help to relax our bodies completely, but it leads to better sleep patterns as well. It is important, however, to make sure that you do not exercise too close to bed time, as this can have the opposite effect.

Chapter 2 – Choosing the Correct Footwear and Clothing

Picking the correct walking shoes are essential! If you select shoes that do not fit correctly, that hurt your feet or are not flexible enough, you will learn to hate your walking experience.

You will have to end up deciding which shoe will be best for you, although there are a few simple things you should take into consideration when making your choice.

Your walking shoe should:

- Be the correct size. It should also provide the correct support to your feet.

- Be flexible and able to conform to your feet properly.

- Provide sufficient cushioning.

The correct size shoe

Choosing the correct size shoe is paramount. You do not want your foot sliding around in a shoe that is far too big. On the opposite end of the equation, you do not want your toes cramped up in the front of the shoe. Even walking for five minutes with shoes like these can cause damage to your feet.

You will have a fair idea of your correct shoe size. Of course, all manufacturers are different, so be sure to try the shoes on, and perhaps more importantly, walk a fair distance in both of them. If you feel any form of discomfort, try another pair.

Walk down an incline as well as upstairs when trying out the shoes. When walking down an incline, your toes should not move forward at all, and should never touch the front of the shoe. Walking on stairs helps to gauge how much your heels will lift when going uphill. Consider trying a new pair of shoes if your heel moves more than 0,3 centimetres. This indicates that you may suffer from blistering to your heel.

Ideally, there should be around a centimetre between where the toes end and the front of the shoe, allowing for some movement for your foot, very important when travelling down steep gradients. Remember to check the width of the shoe as well. Your toes should be spaciously spread out and not crumpled together because the shoe is not wide enough.

When buying a new pair of walking shoes, it is best to try them on at the end of a long day. At this point your feet will be swollen from your day's activities. Try to take a pair of socks with that you will use during walking, or at least the same kind of thickness.

Flexibility

The shoes that you choose should be fairly flexible. Take then in your hands and twist. Do they bend and flex easily? A good walking shoe should!

Why does a shoe need to be flexible? At the end of the day, it all comes down to comfort. As you take each step, your foot flexes as first the heel, then the middle and finally your toes strike the surface. Your shoe therefore should do the same. If not, the natural motion your foot makes when striking the ground will work against the inflexible shoe and this can lead to shin splints.

Perform this quick check. Take the shoe and twist it. It should twist very easily and come back to its proper shape. Then bend the shoe. Make sure it bends where the ball of your foot would be and not around the middle section of the arch. Finally, place the shoe on the ground and push down on where your front toe would be. Does the shoe rock slightly? If so, then the shoe passes the flexibility test.

Also check to see that the material the shoe is made out of will be able to breathe efficiently, allowing sweat from your feet the chance to evaporate effectively.

Cushioning

As you will be walking fair distances in your shoes, you should ensure that they have the correct cushioning to protect your feet. Luckily, a walking shoe does not require as much cushioning as a running shoe might, but it should still have enough support. The most important areas for cushioning are the heel as well as the ball of the foot as these are first to strike the ground.

Other factors

There are a number of minor factors that you can also consider when purchasing your walking shoes.

- The lighter the shoes the better, especially if you are walking a fair distance.

- Some form of shock absorption (especially in the cushioning), can make the shoes more comfortable.

- Depending on weather conditions in the area that you walk, you may consider buying a shoe that is waterproof.

- Pick shoes with low heels that provide support. Thicker, wider heels often cause the feet to hit the tarmac very hard instead of falling in a nice rolling motion. This results in a loss of momentum and increased irritation on the shins.

- Always try to walk your shoes in by wearing them for a few days around the house before using them for a walking workout.

Although not as important as choosing the correct shoes, there are a number of clothing items that you can consider to enhance your walking experience.

When choosing the correct clothing, these are the aspects you should take into account:

- Socks.

- Clothing for specific weather conditions.

- Accessories

Socks

After shoes, the socks you choose are the most critical aspect of your walking clothes. Socks need to do a number of things. Firstly, they offer a second barrier of protection to your feet after your shoes. Secondly, the sock must be able to allow any perspiration from your feet to evaporate properly. If they are unable to do this, walking will not only be uncomfortable, possibly leading to blisters, but your shoes will end up damaged.

The best socks in this regards are made out of an all-synthetic material. If you go on long walks and suffer with very sweaty feet, you may consider changing your socks fairly often, but especially if they are wet with perspiration.

Socks can also offer padding around the heel and ball of the foot, providing even more comfort.

Clothing for specific weather conditions

As the seasons change, you will be walking in varied weather conditions.

When walking in hot weather, try to wear synthetic fibres that do not absorb sweat. Always aim to wear fairly light colours as these will help to reflect both the light and heat of the sun, leaving you cooler. Wear a hat to prevent sunburn and dehydration.

In cold weather, it is critical to wear layers of clothing to keep the warmth in. Pay particular attention to your exposed body parts such as your hands. The first layer of clothing should be synthetic material to allow any perspiration to evaporate. A second layer should be insulating, helping to ensure that body heat is trapped in. These layers can be wool or light fleece. A zipper on this layer can help control the levels of heat. The third layer is often the outer layer, and should not only be water resistant, but also have the ability to keep the wind out.

Accessories

There are numerous accessories that you can use while walking.

- Sunglasses. These are very important for protecting your eyes, especially in sunny conditions.

- Water bottle/CamelBak. Even if you are only walking for twenty minutes, water is essential to keep you hydrated. For longer walks try to drink water at least every 20 minutes.

- Heart rate monitor. A heart rate monitor can be particularly useful if you are want to keep your heart rate at a constant level, especially when trying to keep a fat burning zone.

- Pedometer. A pedometer is a great little gadget that helps to count all the steps you have made. You should be aiming to build up to around 10 000 steps a day.

- Music. A lot of walkers enjoy the accompaniment of music. You may consider a personal music device to help make the miles fly by!

Chapter 3 – Warm Up Routines

Even though walking is a fairly low impact form of exercise, it is essential that you warm up properly beforehand.

Why should you warm up before a walk? Well a warm up does a number of important things.

- It helps to increase the core temperature of your body. This actually helps you to burn more calories as you exercise. It also will increase your heart rate slightly as well.
- Blood circulation throughout your body is increased. This helps to bring more oxygen to your muscles, essential for the workout ahead.
- It increases your muscle temperature which gives them increased elasticity and flexibility. This can help to prevent injury.

Even if you are just starting out in your working program, you MUST warm up!

An ideal warm up

A warm up does not need to be very long. It can include some basic exercises followed by some stretches.

Let's take a closer look at a few basic exercises that you should make part of your pre-walk warm up. These will target both the movements and muscles that form part of the process of walking. You can do each of these exercises for at least 45 seconds prior to starting your walk.

- Ankle warm up. While standing on one leg, flex the ankle of your raised foot in a circular motion. Make sure you move it through a full circle, at least 8 times, first to the right and then to the left. Do this for each foot.

- Leg warm up. While standing on one leg, swing your free leg from your hip, first to the front and then to the back. Keep your leg as relaxed as possible. You do not need to swing it very high, just keep it moving in a relaxed, pendulum type motion. Do 20 swings for each leg.

- Hip warm up. Stand with your knees slightly bent and your feet a shoulder width apart. Place your hands on your hips. While keeping your body as straight as possible, move your hips in circular motion at a slow pace. Do this for 10 circles. Once you have finished with the first set, do the same hip circles in the opposite direction.

- Arm warm up. Place your arms straight out at 90 degrees to your side. Move them in a circular motion, starting out with small movements and gradually increasing the size of the circles. Begin with your hands and as the circles increase in size, end with your whole arm. Do this 12 times, first clockwise and then anti-clockwise.

Remember to do each of these exercises for at least 45 seconds prior to walking. Try to warm up for three minutes in total. If you plan on walking fairly fast, you can do them for slightly longer to ensure that all your muscles are warmed up properly.

Can stretching be incorporated?

Stretching is an extremely good way to ensure that your muscles are flexible and it also helps you to walk comfortably, without pain or stiffness. Stretching should only ever be undertaken once you have completed the warm ups described above. This ensures that the muscle groups have done a range of motions and ultimately helps in the prevention of injuries.

There are a number of quick and easy stretches that you can perform before starting out. These will need to be performed with the help of a chair, so you probably want to do them at home. If you are not able to do them, ensure that your muscles have warmed up properly using the routines described earlier in the chapter.

- Ankle, hamstring and thigh stretches. Place your chair in an empty space and sit on the edge of it. Extend your right leg, making sure that the heel is on the floor. The heel must be flat, so do not extend it too far. Keep your toes pointed while flexing your foot. As you do this, lean slightly forward from your hips until you feel a slight stretching in your thigh, hamstring and ankle. Hold this position for a count of five. Relax and repeat. Do this three times and then swap to your left leg.

- Calf stretches. Stand tall while holding onto the chair. First place your left leg behind you but be sure to keep the heel flat on the floor. Now bend your right knee while leaning slightly towards the chair. As you do this you will feel your calf muscle in your left leg begin to stretch. Hold this position for a count of five. Relax and repeat. Do this three times and then swap to your right leg.

- Groin stretches. Stand behind the chair while holding onto it. Place your legs apart, just a little more than the width of your shoulders. Your left foot should now face forward while you point your right foot at a 45 degree angle to the right. Now lunge forward. Do not let your knee move past your toes. Hold this position for a count of five. Relax and repeat. Do this three times and then swap to your left leg.

Now that you are properly warmed up and your muscles have been sufficiently stretched, it's time to get to the business of walking!

Chapter 4 –   A 10,000 Step

Walking Program

10,000 steps! You have heard this all before. 10,000 steps is what you should aim for each day to reap all the true benefits that walking can offer you.

The truth is, if you are a senior citizen, very unfit or obese, 10,000 steps is not in your range... yet. Look at it this way. If you are inactive, any amount of exercise is going to be beneficial to your health. That is a fact!

But let's say you get to a point where you are getting fitter or maybe you have lost a large amount of weight and you want to push onto those 10,000 steps a day. Well, that's great and it is something you should be encouraged to do. 10,000 steps actually equates to around 30 minutes of exercise or 5 miles of walking.

The history of 10,000 steps

How exactly did this number come about?

Well, it is believed that the 10,000 step phenomena actually started out in Japan. In the 1960's, pedometers became very popular in that country. They were marketed under the name

"Manpokei", which when translated to English means "10,000 steps metre". And so the legend of the 10,000 steps a day was born!

The average person only walks around 4000 - 5000 steps a day, so you will have to double the amount of steps you take to reach this magical figure!

How exactly do you go about it?

Start slowly

Reaching your target will not happen overnight but there are a few simple things you can put in place to start to increase the amount of steps you take each day. Here are a few basic ideas.

- Choose the furthest parking bay away from the entrance of the mall, your work or local store.

- Take a walk around your office during lunch. Even better, venture outside for a nice stroll.

- Instead of using a lift, take the stairs.

That's just the start. Follow the steps below reach your goal.

Building up to 10,000 steps

These five steps will help you reach your goal in next to no time at all!

- Purchase a pedometer. This is the best way to count the steps you make. You don't need anything fancy. You can purchase one that attaches to your clothing or your shoes. If you want to track even more information, a fitness tracker can count your steps, calculate calories burned and even track distance travelled.

- Log your progress. By tracking your daily steps you have a record to look back on and see the progress you have made. Research has shown that people who keep a record of their activities tend to stay motivated for longer. Use a method that works for you, be it paper and pen, an electronic spreadsheet or even a whiteboard.

- Count your steps. You need to find out how many steps you do on average each day. When you know this amount, you will then be able to put your plan into action.

- Increase your steps. Once you know how many steps you walk a day, try to increase it by at least 20 percent over the course of a week. If you walk 5000 steps a day, try to increase it to 6000 steps.

- Continue the process. Follow this procedure each week, increasing the amount of steps you take by 20%, until you reach the 10,000 step mark.

A word of warning

Do not push yourself too far! Listen to your body and if you feel any discomfort at all, either in your muscles or possibly pains in your chest, STOP!

If you suffer from any health issues, it is important that you speak with your doctor before undertaking any strenuous walking.

Chapter 5 – Strolling, Fitness Walking/ Power Walking

As we discovered in Chapter 1, walking has numerous physical, health and mental benefits. How exactly do we get the maximum out of a walk to gain all of these benefits?

The good news is that it is totally up to you! You know exactly why you are walking and there could be a multitude of reasons. Maybe you are walking to lose some extra weight you have gained? Perhaps walking will help you relieve stress from your daily life or maybe you just want to get a little more active and increase your fitness levels.

Once you know exactly why you are walking, then you can decide how you want to attack your walking schedule. The most important thing to understand is that no form of walking be it a stroll or fitness/power walk, is better than the other. ALL walking is good for you!

The leisurely stroll

If you are unfit, or haven't walked long distances in a long time, this is the way that you want to start out. You may be obese and walking is the form of exercise you have chosen to help you to lose weight. You might even be a senior citizen and decided that walking will help to benefit your health.

In these scenarios, you are never going to be a power walker. You want to start out slowly, even 5 minutes a day and build up over time, eventually reaching a fitness level, extended walking time and a pace that you are happy with.

Fitness/Power walking

Fitness or Power walking is a much more vigorous form of exercise which aims to include the muscles of your upper body during the walk. This form of walking is a perfect aerobic activity, good for raising your heart rate and burning calories. Fitness walking is also a great way to achieve muscle tone in the abs, upper back, shoulders, hips, thighs and buttocks.

When walking in this manner, it is important to keep a brisk pace and to swing your arms to increase aerobic activity. Do not swing them too vigorously, just try to keep them in rhythm with each step. Never wear weights on your arms as this may lead to tendon damage.

During fitness walking, all movements are more vigorous and intense. Your stride will be longer than when you walk normally and more often than not will be undertaken at a much quicker pace. Ensure that your shoes have proper cushioning as your heel will strike the ground much harder than it would during a normal walk.

Fitness walking is undertaken specifically as a way to increase one's physical fitness over time.

How to increase your walking speed

When you start your walking routine, you will probably start as a stroller. As you increase your fitness level you may choose to try fitness/power walking. How exactly do you learn to build up your speed to help you reach this level? Following these simple steps will help.

- Always focus on maintaining good posture. Keep your frame as tall as possible. Do not look down at the ground. Try to maintain eye contact on a position around 6 metres ahead of you. Keep your head as straight as possible and your chin level.

- Always keep your shoulders as relaxed as possible.

- Always keep your chest raised.

- Always keep your arms bent at around an 80 degree angle. At the same time, cup your hands. Never let your arms cross your body as you walk. They should only swing from side to side. Your elbows should never pass higher than three-quarters of the way up your chest (in line with your sternum bone).

- Always tighten your buttocks and your abs as you walk. Try to keep your back as flat as possible and push your pelvis out and forward.

- Decide on a step pattern. Some people prefer shorter, faster steps while others prefer to stride out. Use what works best for you.

- Focus on your steps. Firstly on your heel and how it lands, aiming to roll through the step motion and finally pushing off on your toes. Your calf muscles will help to push you forward as you walk.

- As you walk, breathe as naturally as possible while trying to take as much oxygen in as you can. If you can talk naturally while walking, your pace is perfect. If you are struggling to speak, you are probably walking too fast.

Chapter 6 – Cool Down Routines

So you have finished your walk and now you are ready to get on with your daily activities. All good and well, but you must not forget how critical a proper cool down period is, especially if you have had a long strenuous walk.

Why is a cool down period essential? Well, after a period of activity, your muscles become tired and actually start to break down slightly. A cool down routine helps to encourage both tissue and muscle repair, builds strength and encourages overall muscle recovery.

Follow these simple cool down routines to help get your body ready for your next workout.

- Cool down period. It is essential just to take some time at the end of your walk to slow your pace down, allowing your body to readjust from its period of heightened activity to a more restful state. This helps the body begin to simulate the state it will experience after you have finished your walk.

  If you have had a strenuous walk and you suddenly stop, your blood will begin to pool in your legs. This can lead to a sudden lowering of your blood pressure and it is at this time that you may feel dizzy or even faint due to a lack of blood to the brain. Try to slow down for a period until you notice breathing patterns returning to normal and your heart rate dropping.

- Stretch. A period of stretching after you walk can be just as beneficial as your pre-walk stretch. Your muscles are now more elastic and therefore much more pliable. By stretching your muscles, you help to relax them and ease any tension out of them that might have built up during your walk. A post-walk stretch also helps to eliminate muscle pains in your calves, hamstrings and quads. A good stretch will also ensure proper blood circulation to your muscles post exercise and help the healing process as muscles break down.

  You could follow the warm-up stretching routine we discussed in Chapter 3 or you could develop your own set of stretches, but be sure to focus on your quads, hamstrings and calves. Try to stretch for a period of at least five minutes in total.

- Keep hydrated. As you exercise you release water from your body in the form of sweat. While hydration is very necessary during exercise, you should also ensure that your body remains hydrated afterwards. This will actually ensure your muscles do not become too sore and will help to increase both muscle flexibility and strength.

How much liquid should you drink? There is a basic principle you can follow. Weigh yourself before you exercise and then again afterwards. There should be a difference and that difference will be water loss. Drink that weight in liquid and around another 50 percent as you will lose some when you urinate. Obviously, this only really counts for a long, vigorous walk and not a 10 minute stroll!

Conclusion

Thank you again for buying this book!

I hope it will provide you with all the information you need to help start a walking program that will benefit you!

The next step is for you to apply what you have learnt in the book and put it into practice. From your first walking session, you will begin to see the numerous benefits that it offers.

Finally, if you enjoyed this book, then I'd like to ask you for a favour, would you be kind enough to leave a review for this book on Amazon? It would be greatly appreciated!

Thank you and good luck!